The Beginner's Guide to Making Bath Bombs

Written by Erica Anderson

<u>Disclaimer:</u>

Contents

Bath bombs aren't a necessity, but they are one of the niceties that makes life more tolerable…

-My good friend Eleanor

What Are Bath Bombs?

Bath bombs, also known as fizzies, are products that can be added to your bathtub (and sometimes your shower) that permeate the room with amazing fragrances and fill the tub with beneficial oils. Bath bombs start fizzing and creating bubbles when they come in contact with water, due to a reaction between the baking soda and citric acid used to create them. The reaction can be calming and soothing if you're sitting in a tub into which a bath bomb has been placed.

You can make a number of different shapes and sizes of bath bombs, and the only limit is your imagination when it comes to finding new molds. While the selection of molds designed specifically for bath bombs is rather limited, you can use any plastic, rubber or silicon mold, regardless of whether or not it's designed for bath bombs.

Bath bombs are available commercially, but there are several reasons you should make your own at home. The first reason is cost, as high-end bath bombs can run you as much as $10 to $15 per bath bomb. Make the same bath bomb at home and you're looking at spending a dollar or two on supplies. Of course, there are cheaper bath bombs on the market, but many of them use sub-par ingredients and contain chemical fragrances instead of essential oils. Homemade bath bombs can be made from completely natural substances that are good for your skin and your health. When you make your own bath bombs, you have ultimate control over what goes into them and you know you aren't needlessly exposing your body to harmful chemicals.

There are a ton of different recipes you can use to make bath bombs, a number of which are contained in later chapters of this book. While this guide is designed with the beginning bath bomb maker in mind, there's more than enough information and recipes that even the most experienced of bath bomb makers should feel they've got their money's worth.

Bath bombs can be made for personal use, but once you get good at making them, you can give them out as gifts to your close friends and family. They can also be made and sold, both online and in person. Given enough time, you might be able to turn your home hobby into a source of extra income. At the very least, you should be able to make enough money to offset the cost of supplies.

Gathering Supplies

Before we get started, you're going to need to gather some supplies. The nice thing about making bath bombs is the supplies you need to start out aren't expensive and you can purchase most of the items at your local grocery store or supermarket. The rest of the items can be acquired online or at your local pharmacy or health food store. The exact ingredients you need will depend on which of the many recipes you plan on making, so hold off on buying all of your supplies until you've read through the book at least once. That way, you'll be able to pick up everything you need in a single trip.

Here are the supplies you're going to need in order to get started:

- Baking soda.
- Citric acid.
- Corn starch.
- A mold.
- Water or witch hazel.

These are the only ingredients you need in your bath bombs, and even the corn starch is optional, as long as you aren't worried about your bath bombs floating at the top of the tub. Let's take a closer look at the ingredients used to make bath bombs.

Baking Soda

This one's easy.

You probably already have a box of baking soda sitting somewhere around the house. If not, you can pick one up for a couple bucks at your local grocery store. It'll be in the baking supplies section. Baking soda, also known as sodium bicarbonate, is one of the two key ingredients in bath bombs that cause them to fizz when they're added to water. The other ingredient is citric acid, which we'll get to in bit.

Baking soda is a chemical salt that's commonly used as a leavening agent for baked goods. When combined with an acid, it undergoes a chemical reaction that creates carbon dioxide. When used for baking, this chemical reaction causes dough to rise. In bath bombs, baking soda reacts with citric acid to create carbon dioxide bubbles that fill the tub and cause the bath bomb to bounce around.

Don't get baking soda confused with baking powder. The two compounds are similar, but baking powder shouldn't be used in bath bombs. Baking powder is made from baking soda, but has added drying and acidifying agents that aren't needed in bath products.

Baking soda is usually mixed with citric acid in bath bomb recipes in a 2:1 baking soda to citric acid ratio. What this means is you use 2 parts baking soda for every 1 part citric acid used. If you were to use 2 cups of baking soda, you would use 1 cup of citric acid.

Citric Acid

As far as acids are concerned, citric acid is a relatively weak acid. It occurs naturally in citrus fruits and is produced commercially by feeding sugar to a mold known as *Aspergillus niger*. It's usually sold in powder form, which is the form you need for bath bombs, and is a white, crystalline powder.

Citric acid can be purchased from a number of locations. Some grocery stores carry it in their baking aisle because some recipes call for it. Your local craft store, pharmacy, health food store and even some beer- and wine-making supply stores will carry it as well. It's also available online and can be purchased in bulk amounts if you're planning on making a lot of bath bombs.

Food grade citric acid is usually more expensive than non-food grade citric acid. If you don't plan on using it for cooking, go with one of the suppliers that sell non-food grade citric acid and you'll save money.

If you aren't able to source citric acid, cream of tartar is considered an acceptable alternative. It's more potent than citric acid, so cut the amount of cream of tartar down to half of the amount of citric acid the recipe calls for. Bath bombs made using cream of tartar won't have the same rapid fizzing action as those made from citric acid, but it'll work in a pinch.

A Mold

You're going to need some sort of mold into which you can press the bath bomb to compact the material and keep it together. The mold determines the shape of the final product. If you've ever seen bath bombs that are shaped like ducklings or kittens or any of a number of other interesting shapes, it's because they were packed into a mold that was shaped like the product you saw.

Some craft stores sell bath bomb molds that are specifically designed for making bath bombs, but the molds you have to choose from are going to be limited. The good news is you can use almost anything you can pack a bath bomb into as a mold.

Here are just some of the many items I've seen used to make bath bombs:

- **Baking molds.**
- **Candy molds.**
- **Egg cartons.**
- **Ice cube trays.**
- **Muffin tins.**
- **Plastic eggs.**
- **Silicon molds.**
- **Silly putty containers.**

When adding the bath bomb mixture to a mold, pack it in a little bit at a time and compress it as much as you can. Bath bombs that aren't packed tightly are prone to falling apart and will crumble before you're able to use them. Even if they make it into the tub, they'll break apart too quickly and will disappear in a quick puff of bubbles.

Properly-packed bath bombs will last a long time in the tub, dancing around and throwing bubbles. The key is packing a little bit at a time and really compacting it and then adding more and more until the mold is full.

Other Supplies

Along with a bit of cornstarch to help hold things together and to help the bath bombs float, the previous 3 items are the only items you're absolutely going to need to create bath bombs. While you could theoretically combine 2 parts baking soda to 1 part citric acid and 1 part cornstarch and add a little moisture to create a bath bomb, you'd be left with a bath bomb that's unscented and is pretty boring. The rest of the ingredients are all optional, but they're the items that give bath bombs their fragrances, their colors and some can even be added to provide health benefits.

The following ingredients can all be added to bath bombs to add a little character:

- **Butters and carrier oils.**
- **Dried flower petals.**
- **Essential oils.**
- **Food coloring.**
- **Herbs and spices.**

The key to adding other ingredients to bath bombs is to only add them in small amounts. You don't want to add so many other ingredients that they throw off the 2:1 baking soda to citric acid ratio. You'll end up with a bath melt instead. Your bombs will still melt in the tub and fill it with great fragrances and beneficial oils, but you won't get the fizzing action most people expect from their bath bombs. When trying new recipes, it takes a bit of experimentation to find the right balance between the other ingredients and the baking soda and citric acid.

Butters and Carrier Oils

Butters and carrier oils are similar in terms of texture and composure, but they serve different purposes when added to bath bombs. They're both made up of fatty oils, but butters are typically solids, while carrier oils may or may not be solid at room temperature. Some carrier oils and butters, like coconut cream and coconut oil, are solid at cooler temperatures, but will melt when temperatures start to rise. It's important to know which of your ingredients are going to melt because if you use too much of those ingredients, your bath bombs will become a gooey mess when the ambient temperature inside your house climbs above the butter's melting point.

Butters are typically added to bath bomb recipes to help solidify them and keep them together. They're good for adding moisture to the skin and may serve a handful of other skin care purposes. They're completely optional when it comes to bath bombs, but are a common ingredient in many recipes.

The following butters can be used in bath bombs:

- **Almond butter.** Almond butter is similar to sweet almond oil, but it's thicker. It's best when used on dry skin, but will serve most skin types well.
- **Aloe vera butter.** This butter is made by blending oil taken from the aloe vera plant with other butters. Aloe vera butter has moisturizing and regenerative properties that make it a good choice for people with damaged skin. It's a

greasy butter, so it's best to use it in small quantities when adding it to bath melts.

- **Apricot kernel butter.** If you've got dry or normal skin, this highly-moisturizing butter may be a good choice. Those with oily skin would probably be better-served choosing one of the other butters. Apricot kernel butter adds a light, nutty fragrance to the bath when it's used in bath bombs.

- **Avocado butter.** This is another butter you want to go light on in your bath bombs because it's so greasy. When used in smaller amounts, it has moisturizing properties and may provide some protection from damaging UV rays.

- **Cocoa butter.** Cocoa butter is the most popular butter used in bath bomb recipes, partially because of its many benefits, but mainly because it adds the faint fragrance of chocolate to the products it's added to. It's derived from the fatty acids of cocoa seeds and carries with it skin softening and moisturizing properties. Cocoa butter works well for most skin types, but is especially beneficial to those who have dry skin or skin that's been damaged by eczema or too much exposure to the sun. Fragrance-free cocoa butter is available for those looking to add the benefits of cocoa butter to their products without adding the smell of chocolate.

- **Coconut cream.** This oil is often used by people with acne and works well for most skin types. It's a solid when the weather is cool, but will liquefy when it gets warm. It adds the slight fragrance of coconut to bath bombs it's added to.

- **Coffee bean butter.** If you like the aroma of coffee, this soft, fragrant butter is a great choice. It has a soft, silky feel and is completely caffeine-free. Coffee bean butter will melt when temperatures start to rise, so use it in small amounts.
- **Hemp butter.** While hemp butter is derived from the cannabis sativa plant, there's no THC in the butter and it's considered safe for use and non-intoxicating. Hemp butter works well for all skin types and is one of the better oils for irritated and inflamed skin.
- **Illipe butter.** Most people haven't heard of Illipe butter, which is derived from the seeds of the Illipe tree, native to Borneo. It's a moisturizing butter that has a higher melting point than most butter, so it's added to bath bombs to firm them up. This butter is best-used in small amounts.
- **Mango butter.** Made from mango seeds, mango butter is rich and creamy. It helps protect the skin from UV damage and is packed full of antioxidants.
- **Shea butter.** Shea butter comes from the nuts of the Shea tree. It's got anti-inflammatory and healing properties and is a good choice for dry and/or inflamed skin. It's one of the few butters that doesn't leave an oily residue behind on the skin.

Carrier oils are plant-based oils that are used to carry essential oils into the skin. Some carrier oils also act as emulsifying agents that disperse essential oils into the bath. Carrier oils should be used in small amounts in bath bombs because they can leave an oily residue both in the tub and on your skin when larger amounts are used. A little bit of carrier oil goes a long way.

The following list contains some of the more common carrier oils:

- **Almond oil.** This inexpensive oil is one of the better carrier oils for use in bath bombs. It works well on all skin types and has regenerative properties. Don't use almond oil if you have nut allergies because it can touch off an allergic reaction. Make sure you label products that contain this oil.
- **Anise oil.** If you like black licorice, you'll love the smell of this fragrant carrier oil. Use it in small amounts, as it can overpower other fragrances in the bath bombs it's added to.
- **Apricot kernel oil.** This carrier oil can be used to ensure essential oils are absorbed into the skin. It's full of beneficial compounds and is a good oil for sensitive skin. There are some people who are allergic to apricot oil, so make sure you add a warning label to products you're selling that contain this oil.
- **Argan oil.** Argan oil is expensive, but it's a great oil for sun-damaged skin. All you need is a small amount of argan oil to realize its benefits.

- **Avocado oil.** While avocado oil will work well with most skin types, it really comes into its own for those who have dry and damaged skin. Unrefined avocado oil smells like avocadoes. Refined avocado oil eliminates the smell while still managing to keep most of the beneficial compounds intact.
- **Castor oil.** Castor oil disperses the compounds in the bath bomb throughout the water column in the tub. Only use a small amount for best results.
- **Coconut oil.** Unrefined coconut oil features the light smell of coconut and is a good emollient oil. Unless you really hate the smell of coconuts, it's best to stick to unrefined coconut oil. Coconut oil is a solid when temperatures are cool, but will melt when they start to climb. Don't count on coconut oil to hold bath bombs together!
- **Grapeseed oil.** Grapeseed oil is an inexpensive oil that's readily absorbed into the skin. It's one of the few carrier oils that doesn't leave a greasy residue behind.
- **Jojoba oil.** It's more expensive than some of the budget oils, but jojoba oil is a great protective oil because it creates a barrier between the skin and the elements. Use small amounts of jojoba oil for best results.
- **Olive oil.** Extra-virgin olive oil is a decent carrier oil that can be used in small amounts in bath bombs.

Carrier oils should be added in small enough amounts to where they're beneficial and will disperse essential oils and other compounds into the water, but you have to be careful not to use too much or the quality of the bath bomb will suffer. You'll know you used too much when you toss a bath bomb in the tub and it doesn't fizz and bubble or if your bath bomb starts to melt when the temperatures in the room rise.

Aromatic Compounds

There are two types of aromatic compounds people use to add fragrances to bath bombs. Synthetic fragrances are chemical compounds that smell great, but have no therapeutic benefits. They're derived in a laboratory and are chemically formulated to mimic smells found in nature. Synthetic oils are common in commercial bath bombs, but most people who make them at home go with more natural fragrances because there are a number of health concerns associated with some chemical fragrances.

Those looking to go all-natural with their bath bombs should use essential oils instead. Essential oils are oils that are contained within plants that give them their characteristic smell. If you want to see essential oils in action, bend an orange peel back and forth and watch the peel closely. You'll see little geysers of oil spray out of the peel and will instantly smell a strong citrus fragrance. The little geysers you see are essential oils erupting from the peel. Other well-known fragrances that can be attributed to essential oils are the smell of eucalyptus trees, mint plants, flowers, and the smell of popular herbs and spices.

When you purchase essential oils, you're buying concentrated amounts of these oils, and it may have taken hundreds, if not thousands of plants to fill the little vial you're holding in your hand. Be aware that essential oils don't just smell good; they're powerful compounds that carry with them a number of benefits, as well as some inherent dangers. While most people can tolerate small amounts of certain essential oils in a bathtub, there is a small percentage of the population who will react negatively when exposed to essential oils. It's important to test them on a small area of your skin to see if you're allergic prior to jumping into a bathtub into which you've placed a bath bomb containing essential oils. Essential oils can cause reactions when used in conjunction with some medications and they may cause some medical conditions to worsen, so always consult with your physician prior to adding essential oils to your daily routine.

Here are just some of the many types of essential oils people use to add fragrance and therapeutic benefits to their bath bombs:

- **Herbal oils.** These oils smell like the fragrant herbs used for cooking. A number of herbal oils can be used in bath bombs, but be careful. Some oils like oregano oil are "hot" oils that can burn the skin when applied topically.
- **Chamomile essential oil.** Adds a fruity, herbaceous fragrance. Roman chamomile and German chamomile are readily available and can be used to soothe dry, damaged skin.
- **Citrus oils.** There are a number of citrus oils available, including lemon, lime, orange and grapefruit. These oils add the fresh scent of citrus to the bath and are energizing and refreshing.
- **Wood oils.** These oils are obtained from the branches and heartwood of trees. They have exotic fragrances and carry a number of therapeutic benefits.
- **Floral oils.** Derived from the petals and buds of flowers, floral oils smell strongly of the flower they're derived from. Some floral oils like

lavender oil are inexpensive, while others like rose oil will cost you a small fortune. The cost of the oil is usually directly related to how easy it is to obtain the oil from the flower.

- **Mint oils.** These oils add the fragrance of mint to bath bombs. They tend to be powerful oils, so use them with caution.

There are some essential oils that are unsafe and shouldn't be used in bath bombs or skin care products. Always, and I mean always, research the oils you're planning on using prior to hopping into a tub containing them.

Essential oils can be added individually to bath bombs to make them smell like a single oil, but they're more commonly used as part of an oil blend. You can buy the oils individually and blend them yourself or you can purchase premade oil blends.

Making Bath Bombs

Bath bombs aren't hard to make as long as you follow this one rule. No matter what other ingredients you add, you need to keep the ratio of baking soda to citric acid at 2 parts baking soda to 1 part citric acid. What this means is for every 2 cups of baking soda you use, you're going to need 1 cup of citric acid.

Combine the baking soda and citric acid together and mix it thoroughly before adding anything else to the mix. Break apart any lumps that form while you're combining the two ingredients. One easy way to make sure the baking soda and citric acid are combined and are lump-free is to combine them in a sifter and sift them into a bowl. I've found this method is much easier than dumping both ingredients into a bowl and then trying to break up the lumps.

When adding liquid ingredients like oils and fragrances, it's important to add them a little at a time, or you run the risk of the water in the liquids setting off the reaction between the baking soda and citric acid. I usually add a few drops at a time and then stir them in before adding more. If you do see bubbling, you can sometimes stop the reaction by smothering it with baking soda and citric acid.

When you're done creating the powder blend, it should be moldable and will be the consistency of damp sand. The amount of wet ingredients that need to be added to achieve this consistency can vary from batch to batch, so you'll have to take that into consideration when making your own bath bombs. You've achieved the right consistency when you can squeeze the mixture in your hand and let go and it retains its shape. There's a fine balance between too little water, which will cause the bath bombs to crumble and break apart when they're removed from the molds, and too much water, which will make them so they can't be molded at all.

If the oils and butters aren't enough to get the mixture to the desired consistency, a spray bottle containing water or witch hazel can be used. Set it to the mist setting and lightly mist the mixture. Stir it in and continue misting and stirring until you've reached the consistency you're looking for.

The Basic Bath Bomb Recipe

This recipe is an extremely simple bath bomb recipe that can be used as a jumping off point for future recipes. It calls for use of citric acid, coconut oil and corn starch, along with a little Epsom salt thrown in for good measure, to create a simple bath bomb that won't do much more than soften the water and fizz in the tub.

If you don't have access to citric acid, you can substitute ½ cup cream of tartar for each cup of citric acid you would have used. The coconut oil can be substituted for other carrier oils if you'd like. The Epsom salts are also optional and can be replaced with equal parts cornstarch. You probably won't get much use out of this recipe on its own, but it's a great jumping off point from which you can create future recipes. In fact, I rarely make a bath bomb that doesn't start with this recipe.

Ingredients:

2 cups baking soda
1 cup citric acid
¼ cup Epsom salts
¼ cup corn starch
2 teaspoons water
2 tablespoons coconut oil, melted

Directions:

1. Combine the dry ingredients in a bowl and stir them together until they're thoroughly combined. Break apart any lumps. If you're adding other dry

ingredients, now's the time to add them and stir them in.

2. Melt the coconut oil and whisk it together with the water. If you're adding other wet ingredients, stir them in.

3. Add the oil/water combination to the dry ingredients a few drops at a time and whisk it in. Go slow. You can add several drops at a time in different places in the bowl to speed things up.

4. Once the mixture is the consistency of damp sand, it's ready to be packed into the molds. Add a small amount to the mold, pack it in tightly and then add more. Continue adding and packing until the mold is full.

5. Let the bath bombs sit for a couple hours before removing them from the molds.

6. Remove them from the molds and let them sit overnight in a cool, dry place to finish drying.

7. Store the bath bombs in an airtight container.

Cupcake Bath Bombs

This recipe is similar to the previous recipe, but it packs the bath bombs into cupcake liners and then "frosts" them with real icing. Remember, no matter how tasty they might look, don't take a bite of these cupcakes!

One key difference you might notice between this recipe and the previous one is that the recipe calls for witch hazel instead of water. Witch hazel is an astringent compound extracted from the leaves and bark of a shrub that's native to North America. It's used in folk medicine to treat a number of skin conditions due to its anti-inflammatory and antimicrobial properties. It can be used interchangeably with water in bath bomb recipes, and is preferred by some who say it causes less premature foaming when it's sprayed onto the bath bomb mixture to dampen it.

Ingredients:

2 cups baking soda
1 cup citric acid
½ cup corn starch
2 tablespoons almond oil
10 drops of your favorite essential oil (or oil blend)
A spray bottle containing witch hazel

¼ cup powdered egg whites
3 cups powdered sugar
¼ cup warm water
Optional: Food coloring

Directions:

1. Combine the dry ingredients in a bowl and whisk them together until all the lumps are gone.
2. Combine the almond oil and essential oil, and stir the combination into the dry ingredients slowly.
3. Mist witch hazel onto the mixture and stir it in until it's the consistency of damp sand and can be molded.
4. Line silicon cupcake molds with cupcake liners and press the bath bomb mixture into the molds.
5. Create the frosting by combining the second set of ingredients and beating it until peaks start to form. If the mixture is too thick, add warm water a tablespoon at a time and beat it in until the mixture is the right consistency.
6. Transfer the frosting to a frosting bag and frost the bath bomb "cupcakes."
7. Allow them to dry before storing them. These cupcakes are difficult to store in taller containers because they can't be stacked. Store them in a flat airtight container or bag them up in individual bags instead.

Cinnamon Vanilla Bombs

I wasn't sure what to expect when I combined cinnamon and vanilla into a single bath bomb. I didn't know whether I'd hate it or love it, and I have to admit. The end result surprised me. The two fragrances meld together to create a bath bomb that smells delicious!

For the cinnamon in this recipe, I used strongly-brewed cinnamon tea. I'm not sure if ground cinnamon would work, but suspect it might. Cinnamon oil might work as well, but if you decide to go that route, only use a small amount. It's a hot oil and can burn the skin.

Ingredients:

2 cups baking soda
1 cup citric acid
1 cup corn starch
¼ cup canola oil
2 tablespoons vanilla
2 to 4 tablespoons strong cinnamon tea
Optional: A couple drops of red food coloring

Directions:

1. Combine the dry ingredients and whisk them together. Make sure you remove any lumps.
2. Combine the canola oil, vanilla and cinnamon tea in a bowl and whisk them together. Add the red food coloring and whisk it in, if you're planning on using it.

3. Add the wet ingredients to the dry ingredients slowly and stir them together, until the mixture is the consistency of damp sand and is moldable.
4. Press the mixture into the molds and let them sit for a few hours.
5. Remove the bath bombs from the molds and let them dry overnight.
6. Store them in an airtight container.

Cocoa Butter Bath Bombs

This recipe is simple by design. It combines a handful of ingredients to create a bath bomb that fills the room with the light fragrance of cocoa. It's beneficial to the skin because cocoa butter contains antioxidants that prevent free radical damage and may help protect the skin from sun damage. One thing's for certain. It's a great bath bomb to pop in the tub on those days when you want a long, relaxing soak in a hot tub.

You can try adding essential oils to this recipe if you'd like, but to be completely honest with you, I've never found a fragrance I like more than the base scent.

Ingredients:

2 cups baking soda
1 cup citric acid
1 cup corn starch
¼ cup cocoa butter
A spray bottle full of water

Directions:

1. Combine the dry ingredients and whisk them together. Make sure you remove any lumps.
2. Melt the cocoa butter. Let it cool a bit and slowly stir it into the dry ingredients. Remove any lumps.
3. Mist the mixture with water and whisk the water in until the mixture is the consistency of damp sand and can be molded.

4. Press the mixture into the molds and let them sit for a few hours.
5. Remove the bath bombs from the molds and let them dry overnight.
6. Store them in an airtight container.

Triple Coconut Bath Bombs

Combine coconut oil, coconut extract and coconut cream into a single bath bomb and what do you get? A bath bomb that's packed full of coconut goodness and is sure to please any fan of coconut! This bath bomb smells good on its own, or you can add your favorite essential oils or oil blend to it to make it smell even better.

Be aware that this bomb might get a little soft in warmer temperatures.

Ingredients:

2 cups baking soda
1 cup citric acid
1 cup corn starch
¼ cup Epsom salts
¼ cup coconut oil
2 tablespoons coconut cream
1 tablespoon coconut extract
A spray bottle containing water
Optional: Food coloring
Optional: Essential oils

Directions:

1. Combine the dry ingredients in a bowl and whisk them together until all the lumps are gone.
2. Melt the coconut oil. Add the coconut cream and coconut extract to it and stir them together. Add the essential oils and food coloring at this time, if you plan on using them.

3. Add the wet ingredients to the dry ingredients slowly, stirring them in as you go. If the proper consistency isn't reached, lightly mist water a spray or two at a time onto the mixture and stir it in until the mixture is moldable like damp sand.
4. Press the mixture into the molds.
5. Let the bath bombs sit for a few hours and then pop them out of the molds.
6. Let them dry for a day or two before storing them in an airtight container.

Congestion Busters

If you've got a cold, allergies or some other sort of respiratory condition that has you feeling all clogged up, this bath bomb might be just what you need to break the congestion up and get some relief.

It uses a potent blend of essential oils, so a short soak in the tub is all that's needed. Inhale deeply and the essential oils should provide at least some relief.

Ingredients:

2 cups baking soda
1 cup citric acid
2 tablespoons shea butter
10 drops eucalyptus essential oil
10 drops lavender essential oil
5 drops peppermint essential oil
A spray bottle full of water

Directions:

1. Combine the baking soda and citric acid in a bowl. Break apart any lumps.
2. Melt the shea butter over Low heat. Let it cool a bit and add the essential oils. Stir them in.
3. Add the oil blend to the dry ingredients slowly. Stir it in and break apart any lumps that form.
4. Mist the mixture with water and stir the water in until it's the consistency of damp sand.
5. Press the mixture into your molds and let them sit for a couple hours.

6. Remove the bath bombs from the molds and let them dry overnight.
7. Store them in an airtight container.

Detox Bombs

These bombs contain ginger and seaweed powder in order to help pull toxins from your body and to cleanse and detoxify the skin. They aren't the greatest-smelling bath bombs around, but you can dress them up with your favorite essential oils to mask the smell.

Ingredients:

2 cups baking soda
1 cup citric acid
¼ cup corn starch
¼ cup Epsom salts
2 tablespoons almond oil
1 tablespoon ground ginger
2 tablespoons seaweed powder
10 drops of your favorite essential oil
A spray bottle full of witch hazel

Directions:

1. Combine the dry ingredients in a bowl and whisk them together until all the lumps are gone.
2. Combine the almond oil and essential oil, and stir the combination into the dry ingredients slowly.
3. Mist witch hazel onto the mixture and stir it in until it's the consistency of damp sand and can be molded.
4. Press the mixture into your molds.
5. Let the bath bombs dry for several hours before removing them from the molds.

6. Let them dry overnight before storing them in an airtight container in a cool, dry place.

Double Chocolate Delight

Chocolate lovers will be in second heaven with this bath bomb since it combines cocoa butter and cocoa powder to create a bath bomb that doubles up on the chocolate goodness!

Keep these out of the reach of children. They smell like chocolate and might entice a youngster to try and take a bite. It probably wouldn't hurt them too much, but they won't be happy when they realize they just bit into something that's anything but the sweet chocolate they were expecting!

Ingredients:

2 cups baking soda
1 cup citric acid
½ cup corn starch
¼ cup cocoa butter
3 tablespoons cocoa powder
2 tablespoons shea butter
A spray bottle full of water or witch hazel

Directions:

1. Combine the dry ingredients and whisk them together. Make sure you remove any lumps.
2. Melt the cocoa butter. Let it cool a bit and slowly stir it into the dry ingredients. Remove any lumps.
3. Mist the mixture with water or witch hazel and whisk the water in until the mixture is the consistency of damp sand and can be molded.

4. Press the mixture into the molds and let them sit for a few hours.
5. Remove the bath bombs from the molds and let them dry overnight.
6. Store them in an airtight container.

Dry Skin Relief

This bath bomb takes 3 different moisturizing butters and oils and combines them with lavender and sandalwood essential oil to create a bath bomb that adds moisture to dry skin and smells great. These bath bombs tend to get a little crumbly, so make sure you really pack them into the molds.

Ingredients:

2 cups baking soda
1 cup citric acid
2 tablespoons corn starch
2 tablespoons cocoa butter
2 tablespoons Aloe vera butter
1 tablespoon sweet almond oil
10 drops lavender essential oil
5 drops sandalwood essential oil
Spray bottle full of water or witch hazel

Directions:

1. Combine the dry ingredients in a bowl and whisk them together until all the lumps are gone.
2. Melt the butters and almond oil. Add the essential oils and stir them in.
3. Add the wet ingredients to the dry ingredients slowly, stirring them in as you go. If the proper consistency isn't reached, lightly mist water or witch hazel a spray or two at a time onto the mixture and stir it in until the mixture is moldable like damp sand.

4. Press the mixture into the molds.
5. Let the bath bombs sit for a few hours and then pop them out of the molds.
6. Let them dry for a day or two before storing them in an airtight container.

Oily Skin Relief

While the previous bath bomb was for people with dry skin, this bomb is designed for those who are on the other end of the spectrum. The frankincense, lavender and patchouli essential oils combine to create an astringent blend that helps rebalance sebum production and should help alleviate oily skin.

Ingredients:

2 cups baking soda
1 cup citric acid
¼ cup corn starch
2 tablespoons cocoa butter
1 tablespoon sweet almond oil
10 drops lavender essential oil
5 drops frankincense essential oil
5 drops patchouli essential oil
A spray bottle with water or witch hazel

Directions:

1. Combine the dry ingredients in a bowl and whisk them together until all the lumps are gone.
2. Melt the cocoa butter and stir in the sweet almond oil. Let the mixture cool for a while and add the essential oils and stir them in.
3. Add the wet ingredients to the dry ingredients slowly, stirring them in as you go. If the proper consistency isn't reached, lightly mist water or witch hazel a spray or two at a time onto the

mixture and stir it in until the mixture is moldable like damp sand.

4. Press the mixture into the molds.
5. Let the bath bombs sit for a few hours and then pop them out of the molds.
6. Let them dry for a day or two before storing them in an airtight container.

Green Tea Bath Bombs

Green tea contains a lot of antioxidants that are good for the skin. The tannin in the green tea is believed to tighten the skin and may help reduce wrinkles. It's also good for your hair and may be able to help prevent baldness and reduce hair loss.

When added to bath bombs, green tea adds the relaxing fragrance most people associate with tea time to the tub. This is one of the bath bombs I turn to when it's time to wind down.

Ingredients:

2 cups baking soda
1 cup citric acid
¼ cup Epsom salts
¼ cup corn starch
¼ cup strong green tea
2 tablespoons coconut oil

Directions:

1. Brew the green tea. Add more leaves than you would if you were brewing it to drink. You want it to be on the strong side.
2. Combine the dry ingredients in a bowl.
3. Melt the coconut oil and whisk it and the green tea together.
4. Add the oil/tea mixture to the dry ingredients a little at a time and whisk it in until combined. Keep adding and whisking it in until the bath bomb

mixture is the texture of wet sand. If it starts to foam, keep stirring until it stops.

5. Add a small amount of the mixture to the molds, pack it in tightly and then add more. Continue adding and packing until each mold is full.

6. Let the bath bombs sit for an hour before removing them from the mold.

7. Remove them from the molds and let them sit overnight in a cool, dry place to finish drying.

8. Store the bath bombs in an airtight container.

Lavender Oatmeal Bombs

The oatmeal in this recipe is added to soothe the skin and leave it feeling silky smooth. I've added both lavender essential oil and dried lavender petals to this recipe, but you can make it without the lavender petals if you don't have any on hand.

Ingredients:

2 cups baking soda
1 cup citric acid
¼ cup oats
1 tablespoon olive oil
15 drops lavender essential oil
Dried lavender petals
Witch hazel

Directions:

1. Grind the oats in a blender or spice grinder.
2. Combine the dry ingredients in a bowl and stir them together until they're thoroughly combined. Break apart any lumps.
3. Combine the olive oil and the lavender essential oil. Add it to the dry ingredients a little bit at a time and stir it in. Break apart any lumps that form.
4. Mist witch hazel onto the mixture and stir it in until the mixture is moldable.
5. Press the mixture into your bath bomb molds a little bit at a time.

6. Gently press the lavender petals into the top of each bath bomb.
7. Give them several hours to dry and remove them from the molds.
8. Let them dry overnight before storing them in an airtight container.

Lavender Honey Bombs

I was hesitant when a friend first told me to try adding honey to my bath bomb recipes because I was worried I was going to leave the tub and sticky mess and get out feeling like I was coated in sticky, sweet honey. I'm glad I went ahead and tried it because, as it turns out, honey in bath bombs might make the bomb itself feel a little tacky, but it won't leave you feeling sticky. The honey dissolves in the warm water and you get a nice, relaxing soak in a tub full of antibacterial goodness.

Ingredients:

2 cups baking soda
1 cup citric acid
¼ cup corn starch
¼ cup shea butter
2 tablespoons raw honey
15 drops lavender essential oil
Dried lavender flowers
A spray bottle containing witch hazel

Directions:

1. Combine the dry ingredients in a bowl and stir them together until they're thoroughly combined. Break apart any lumps.
2. Melt the shea butter. Combine the shea butter, honey and the lavender essential oil. Add the mixture to the dry ingredients a little bit at a time and stir it in. Break apart any lumps that form.

3. Mist witch hazel onto the mixture and stir it in until the mixture is moldable.
4. Press the mixture into your bath bomb molds a little bit at a time.
5. Gently press the lavender petals into the top of each bath bomb.
6. Give them several hours to dry and remove them from the molds.
7. Let them dry overnight before storing them in an airtight container.

Lemongrass Citrus Bath Bombs

Lemongrass citrus bath bombs have a refreshing citrus fragrance that provides a pick-me-up on those days you're feeling down in the dumps. I use these bath bombs to reinvigorate myself in the middle of the week when I'm starting to feel burnt out.

Orange zest is created by peeling an orange and then removing the pith from the peel and grating or chopping the remaining portion of the peel into tiny pieces. It contains orange essential oils and will add a light citrus fragrance to any bath bomb it's added to.

Ingredients:

2 cups baking soda
1 cup citric acid
¼ cup corn starch
1 tablespoon olive oil.
2 tablespoons orange zest
10 drops lemongrass essential oil
Spray bottle with witch hazel

Directions:

1. Combine the citric acid, orange zest and baking soda in a bowl. Stir until all of the lumps are gone.
2. Combine the olive oil and the lemongrass essential oil in a bowl and then stir the oil mixture into the dry ingredients, adding a little at a time to prevent foaming.

3. Place the witch hazel into a spray bottle and mist it onto the mixture a little at a time. Stir it in and continue misting and stirring until the mixture is the right consistency.
4. Press it into your bath bomb molds.
5. Allow the bath bombs to dry for a few hours before removing them from the mold.
6. Let them dry overnight before storing them in an airtight container.

Men's Bath Bombs

A number of men I know make the argument that bath bombs are somewhat feminine by nature, and they refuse to use them. My husband was the same way until I crafted this bath bomb and convinced him to try it once. He probably won't be happy I made his use of bath bombs public knowledge (sorry dear!), but he'll get over it. If not, I'll hold back his weekly supply of bath bombs until he does!

The smell of sandalwood and Vetiver combined creates a manly fragrance that most men love. The hard part is convincing them to try it for the first time.

Ingredients:

2 cups baking soda
1 cup citric acid
½ cup Epsom salts
2 tablespoons coconut oil, melted
5 drops Vetiver essential oil
5 drops sandalwood essential oil
Spray bottle full of water

Directions:

1. Combine the dry ingredients in a bowl and whisk them together until all the lumps are gone.
2. Melt the coconut oil. Add the essential oils and stir them in.
3. Add the wet ingredients to the dry ingredients slowly, stirring them in as you go. If the proper consistency isn't reached, lightly mist water a spray

or two at a time onto the mixture and stir it in until the mixture is moldable like damp sand.

4. Press the mixture into the molds.
5. Let the bath bombs sit for a few hours and then pop them out of the molds.
6. Let them dry for a day or two before storing them in an airtight container.

Moisturizing Patchouli Bath Bomb

For those who haven't yet smelled patchouli essential oil, you're in for a special treat. It has an exotic fragrance that may take a bit of getting used to, but once you've smelled it a couple times, you'll probably fall in love with it.

This bath bomb uses a blend of cocoa butter and shea butter for moisturizing. Try adding your favorite citrus oils to the recipe to switch up the smell a bit.

Ingredients:

2 cups baking soda
1 cup citric acid
¼ cup corn starch
2 tablespoons cocoa butter
2 tablespoons shea butter
10 drops patchouli essential oil
A spray bottle full of water (or witch hazel)

Directions:

1. Combine the baking soda, citric acid and corn starch in a bowl. Break apart any lumps.
2. Melt the shea butter and cocoa butter over Low heat. Let it cool a bit and add the patchouli essential oil. Stir it in.
3. Add the oil blend to the dry ingredients slowly. Stir it in and break apart any lumps that form.
4. Mist the mixture with water (or witch hazel) and stir it in until it's the consistency of damp sand.

5. Press the mixture into your molds and let them sit for a couple hours.
6. Remove the bath bombs from the molds and let them dry overnight.
7. Store them in an airtight container.

Oregano Shea Butter Bath Bomb

Oregano essential oil smells just like the herb used for cooking, only stronger. It's strongly-antibacterial and has the power to fight off infections both inside and outside the body. It's said to slow down cellular deterioration, which may slow down the effects of aging.

Oregano oil is considered a hot oil, so make sure you can tolerate it prior to adding it to your bath bombs. Only use a small amount of this potent oil for best results.

Ingredients:

2 cups baking soda
1 cup citric acid
1 cup corn starch
2 tablespoons water
2 tablespoons Shea butter
15 drops oregano essential oil

Directions:

1. Combine the dry ingredients in a bowl.
2. Melt the Shea butter and whisk it together with the water and the oregano essential oil.
3. Add the oil/water mixture to the dry ingredients a little at a time and whisk it in until combined. Keep adding and whisking until the bath bomb mixture is the texture of wet sand.
4. Add a small amount of the mixture to each of the molds, pack it in tightly and then add more.

Continue adding and packing until each mold is full.

5. Let the bath bombs sit for a few minutes before removing them from the mold.
6. Remove them from the molds and let them sit overnight in a cool, dry place to finish drying.
7. Store the bath bombs in an airtight container.

Peppermint Bath Bombs

Peppermint bath bombs don't just fill the room with the refreshing fragrance of peppermint. They're made using peppermint essential oil, which refreshes and invigorates the mind and can be used to clear up congestion due to colds and other respiratory conditions. You'll breathe easier and feel better after adding one of these bath bombs to the tub.

Ingredients:

2 cups baking soda
1 cup citric acid
¼ cup corn starch
2 tablespoons shea butter
5 drops peppermint essential oil
Spray bottle with witch hazel
Optional: Red food coloring

Directions:

1. Combine the dry ingredients in a bowl and stir them together until they're combined. Break apart any lumps.
2. Melt the shea butter and stir in the peppermint essential oil. Add several drops of red food coloring at this time, if you want to color the bath bombs.
3. Add the oil combination to the dry ingredients a few drops at a time and whisk it in. Go slow. You can add several drops at a time in different places in the bowl to speed things up.

4. Mist the mixture with witch hazel and stir it in until it's the right consistency.

5. Once the mixture is the consistency of damp sand, it's ready to be packed into the molds. Add a small amount to the mold, pack it in tightly and then add more. Continue adding and packing until the mold is full.

6. Let the bath bombs sit for a couple hours before removing them from the mold.

7. Remove them from the molds and let them sit overnight in a cool, dry place to finish drying.

8. Store the bath bombs in an airtight container.

Pumpkin Spice Bath Bombs

Here's a great fall gift that smells like a fresh slice of pumpkin pie. Oddly enough, it doesn't have any pumpkin in it. Instead, it relies on an essential oil blend that creates a fragrance similar to that of the spices used to make pumpkin pie.

To make these bath bombs even more festive, round up a cookie cutter or a mold that's shaped like a pumpkin. If you really want to get fancy, you can dye the stems green and the pumpkins orange. Just be sure the dye you're using is safe for your skin (and your tub)!

Ingredients:

2 cups baking soda
1 cup citric acid
1 tablespoon olive oil
½ cup strong cinnamon tea
2 drops nutmeg essential oil
2 drops clove bud essential oil
2 drops cardamom essential oil

Directions:

1. Combine the citric acid and baking soda in a bowl. Stir until all of the lumps are gone.
2. Combine the olive oil and the essential oils in a bowl and stir them into the dry ingredients, adding a little at a time to prevent foaming.
3. Place the cinnamon tea into a spray bottle and mist it onto the mixture a little at a time. Stir it in and

continue misting and stirring until the mixture is the right consistency.

4. Press it into your bath bomb mold. If you're using a cookie cutter, place the cookie cutter on a flat surface and press the mixture into the cookie cutter.

5. Allow the bath bombs to dry for a few hours before removing them from the mold. Let them dry overnight before storing them in an airtight container.

Triple Rose Bath Bombs

Rose essential oil is on the expensive side, but a small bottle of rose oil can be used to create a large number of bath bombs. This recipe calls for three different rose products to be added: the aforementioned rose essential oil, rose petals and rose water.

This triple rose action smells amazing and is calming and sedative. It soothes the mind and is also a great choice for soothing dry, irritated skin. It can make you a bit drowsy, so it's best left for the end of the day.

Ingredients:

2 cups baking soda
1 cup citric acid
¼ cup Epsom salts
½ cup corn starch
2 teaspoons olive oil
7 drops rose essential oil
A spray bottle full of water or witch hazel
Dried rose petals
Optional: A couple drops of red food coloring

Directions:

1. Combine the dry ingredients in a bowl.
2. Whisk the olive oil and rose essential oil together. If you're using red food coloring, add it to the oil mixture and whisk it in. Add the oil mixture to the dry ingredients several drops at a time and whisk it in.

3. If the mixture is too dry, set the spray bottle to mist and lightly mist it with water or witch hazel. Stir the water in and continue misting until the mixture is moldable.
4. Pack the mixture into the molds and let them sit for 15 minutes.
5. Remove the bath bombs from the molds and let them dry overnight.
6. Store the bath bombs in an airtight container.

Storing Bath Bombs

Bath bombs are sensitive to heat, light and moisture, so they need to be stored in an airtight container and kept in a cool, dark place. Plastic or glass containers are preferable because you don't have to worry about chemical reactions taking place where the bath bombs are in contact with the container.

If you're planning on giving bath bombs as gifts or selling them, mason jars are a good storage container. You can seal them in the jar, decorate it with a nice label and/or bow and they're ready to go. Another option is to seal them in a plastic bag, but this isn't as aesthetically pleasing.

www.ingramcontent.com/pod-product-compliance
Lightning Source LLC
Chambersburg PA
CBHW060645290526
45793CB00001B/400